# TABLE OF CONTENT

# INTRODUCTION

"25 Tasty Smoothies for Weight Loss" is a comprehensive guide to the world of healthy and delicious smoothies. In this book, we'll explore the benefits of incorporating smoothies into your diet, as well as provide you with 25 easy-to-follow recipes that are designed specifically for weight loss. Whether you're a seasoned smoothie drinker or new to the world of blended drinks, this book has something for everyone.

Smoothies are a convenient and delicious way to increase your daily intake of fruits and vegetables, and they are also an excellent way to achieve weight loss goals. By replacing high-calorie meals and snacks with healthy smoothies, you can cut calories and enjoy a variety of different flavors and ingredients. Additionally, many of the ingredients used in smoothies, such as leafy greens, are nutrient-dense and can help to boost your overall health and wellbeing.

This book is written for people of all levels of experience, from those who are new to smoothie making to those who have been blending for years. You are going to love the 25 delicious recipes that are designed specifically for weight loss.

# INTRODUCTION

Each recipe in this book is carefully crafted to deliver a delicious, healthy smoothie that will help you achieve your weight loss goals. From classic fruit smoothies to green smoothies and everything in between, you'll find a perfect recipe. Each recipe includes a detailed list of ingredients, easy-to-follow instructions, and helpful tips and tricks for making the perfect smoothie every time.

One of the keys to successful weight loss is variety, and this book has got you covered in that department. Whether you're in the mood for something sweet and fruity, or you're looking for a more savory green smoothie, you'll find a recipe that meets your needs and taste preferences. And, because all of the ingredients used in these smoothies are easily accessible, you can make these drinks anytime, anywhere.

So, if you're ready to start your weight loss journey and enjoy the benefits of healthy, delicious smoothies, then grab a blender and let's get started! With 25 tasty smoothie recipes to choose from, you'll never be bored or run out of ideas. Whether you're a busy professional, a student, or simply someone who is looking for a quick and easy way to improve your diet and reach your weight loss goals, this book has got you covered. So, what are you waiting for? Start blending and enjoy the benefits of delicious smoothies today!

# 01 Strawberry Banana Smoothie

## INGREDIENTS

- 1 banana
- 1 cup frozen strawberries
- 1 cup unsweetened almond milk
- 1 scoop vanilla protein powder
- 1 tsp honey

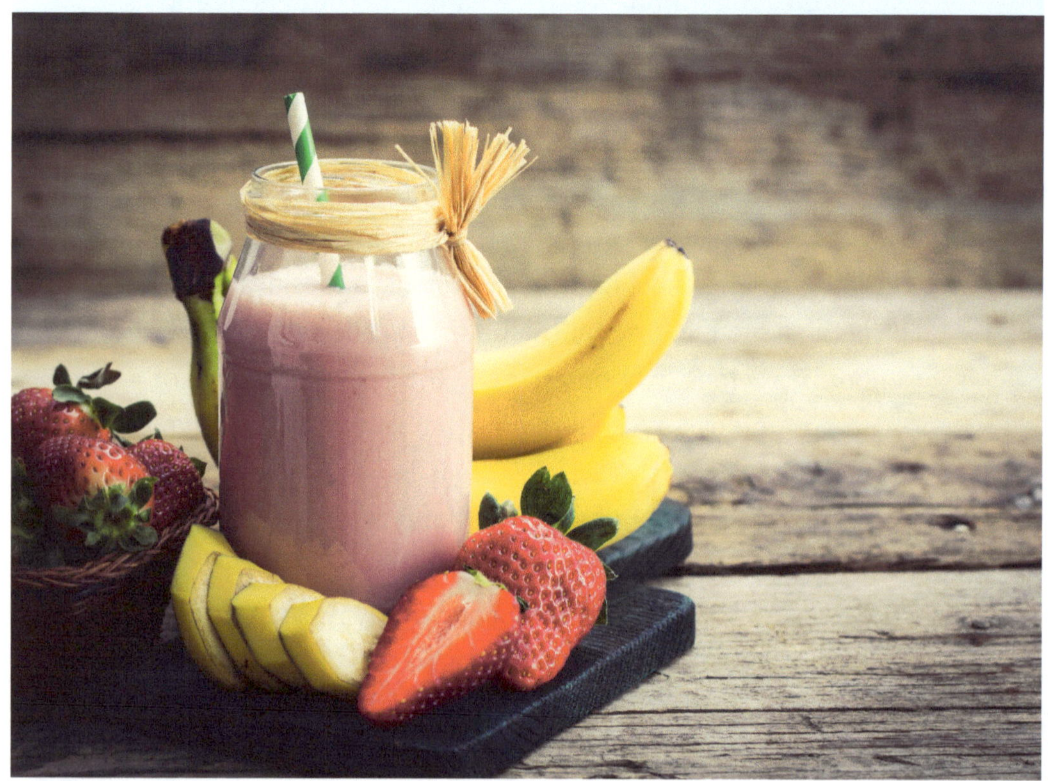

# 02 Green Goddess Smoothie

## INGREDIENTS

- 1 banana
- 1 cup kale
- 1 cup spinach
- 1 cup unsweetened almond milk
- 1/2 avocado
- 1 tbsp lemon juice
- 1 tsp honey
- 1 scoop vanilla protein powder

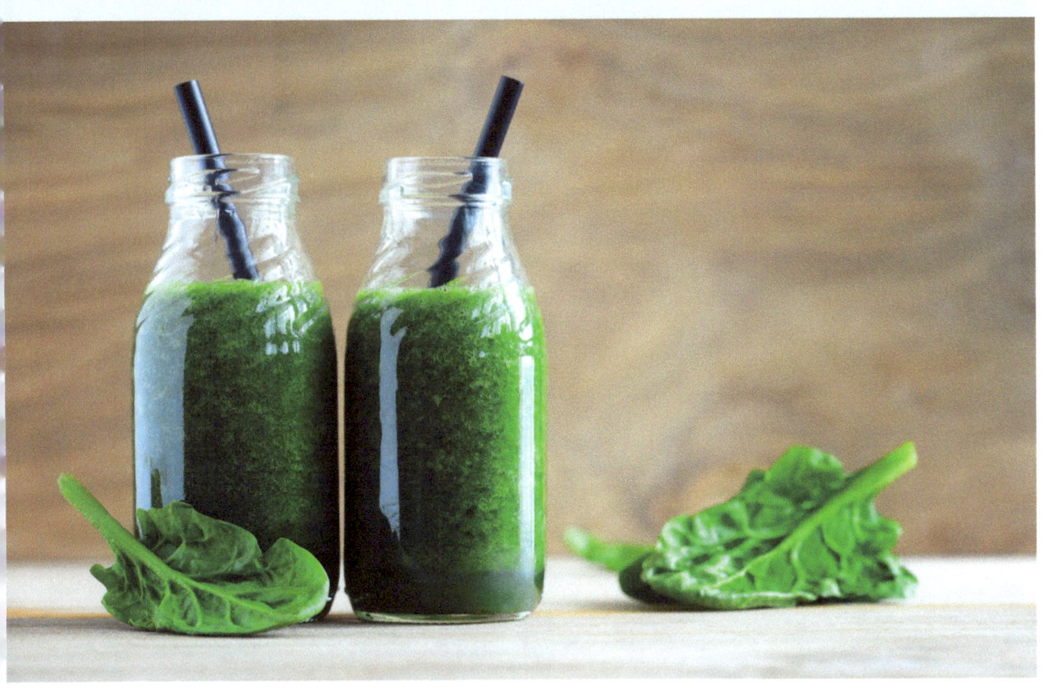

# 03 Blueberry Oat Smoothie

## INGREDIENTS

- 1 cup frozen blueberries
- 1 banana
- 1/2 cup rolled oats
- 1 cup unsweetened almond milk
- 1 scoop vanilla protein powder
- 1 tsp honey

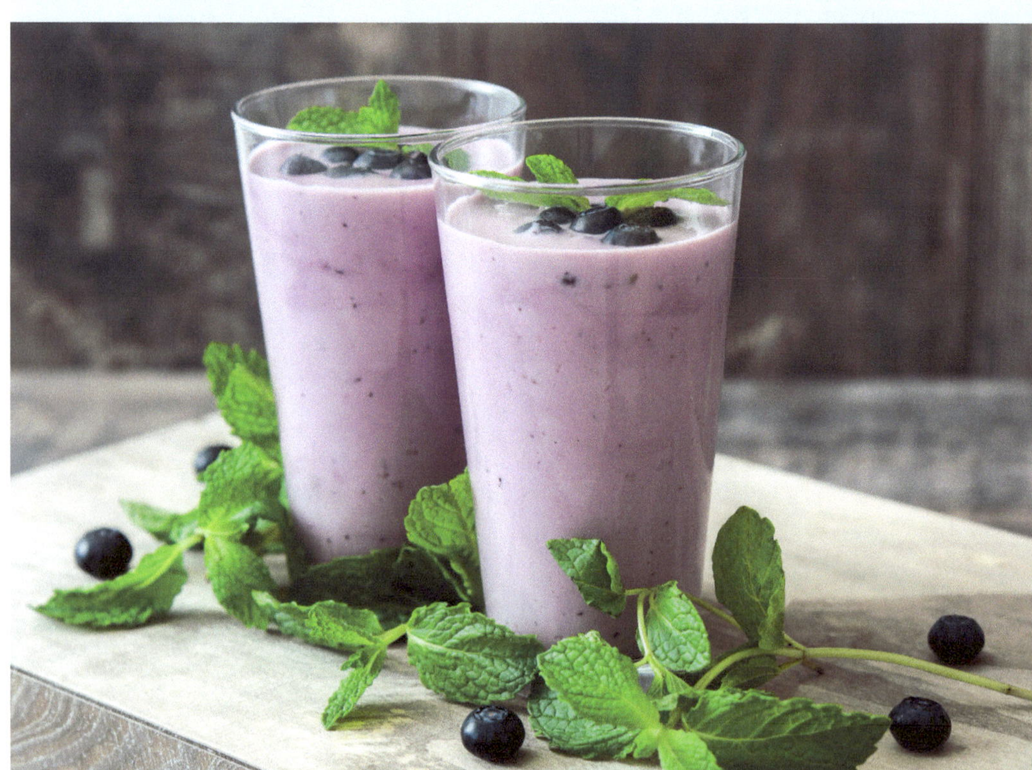

# Mango Ginger Smoothie

**04**

## INGREDIENTS

- 1 cup frozen mango
- 1 banana
- 1 inch piece of fresh ginger
- 1 cup unsweetened almond milk
- 1 scoop vanilla protein powder
- 1 tsp honey

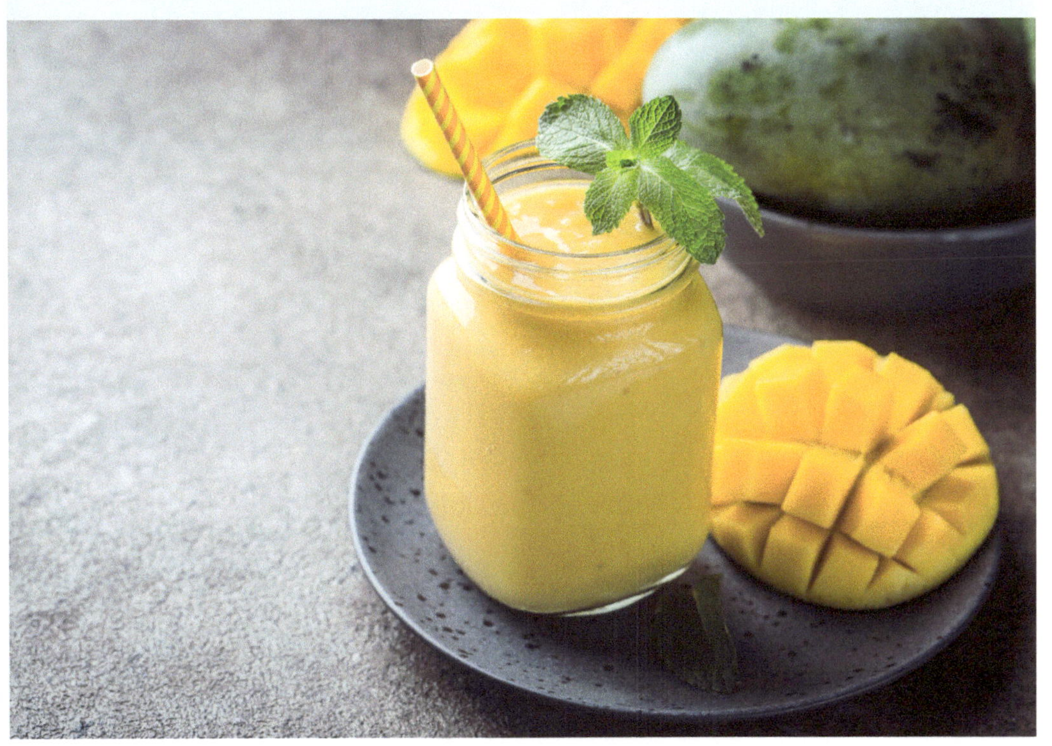

# Peanut Butter Banana Smoothie

**05**

## INGREDIENTS

- 1 banana
- 1 tbsp peanut butter
- 1 cup unsweetened almond milk
- 1 scoop vanilla protein powder
- 1 tsp honey

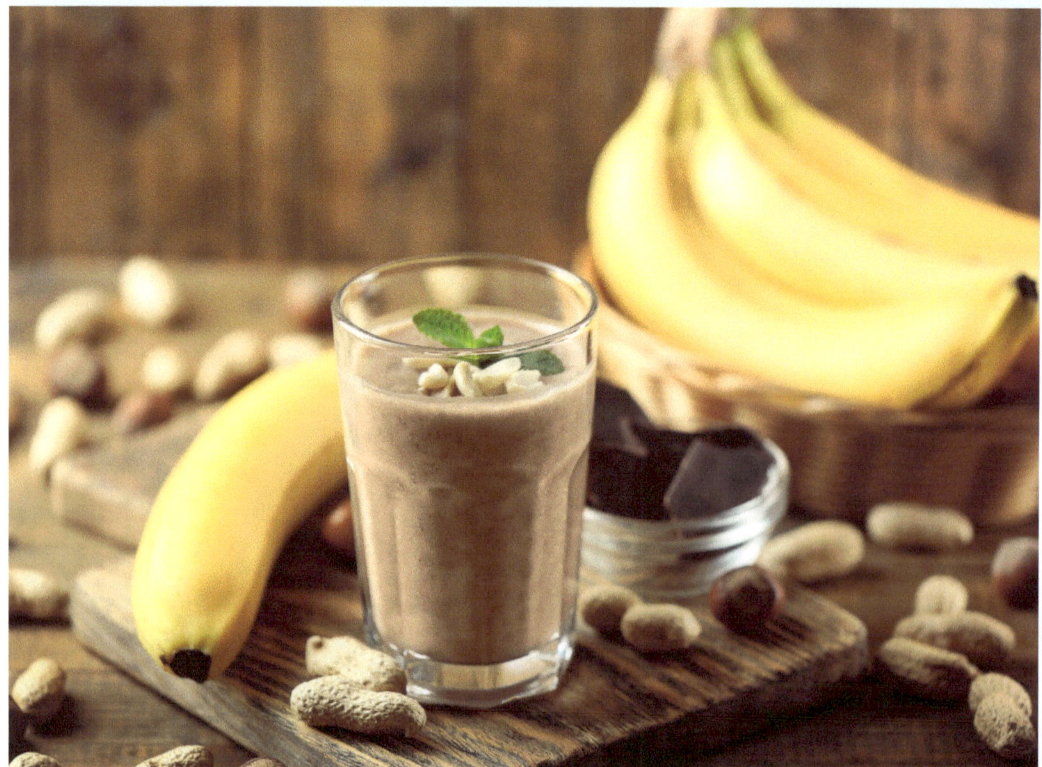

# 06 Pineapple Coconut Smoothie

## INGREDIENTS

- 1 cup frozen pineapple
- 1/2 cup unsweetened coconut milk
- 1 scoop vanilla protein powder
- 1 tsp honey

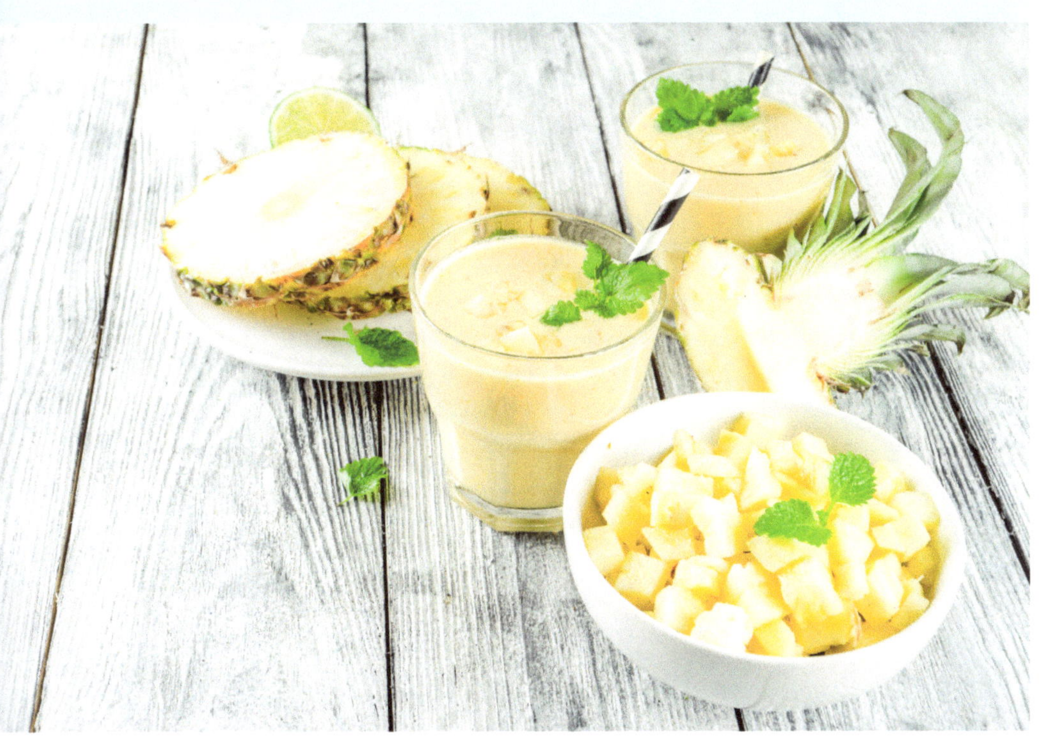

# Chocolate Cherry Smoothie

07

## INGREDIENTS

- 1 cup frozen cherries
- 1 banana
- 1 tbsp cacao powder
- 1 cup unsweetened almond milk
- 1 scoop chocolate protein powder
- 1 tsp honey

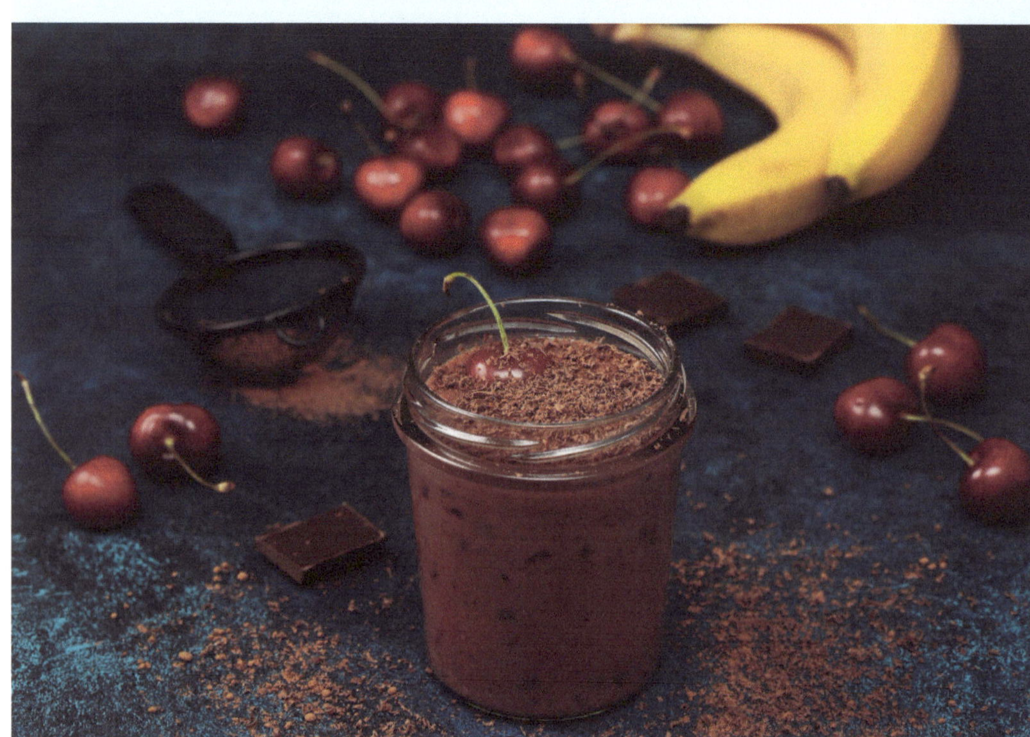

# 08 Raspberry Orange Smoothie

## INGREDIENTS

- 1 cup frozen raspberries
- 1 banana
- 1/2 cup freshly squeezed orange juice
- 1 cup unsweetened almond milk
- 1 scoop vanilla protein powder
- 1 tsp honey

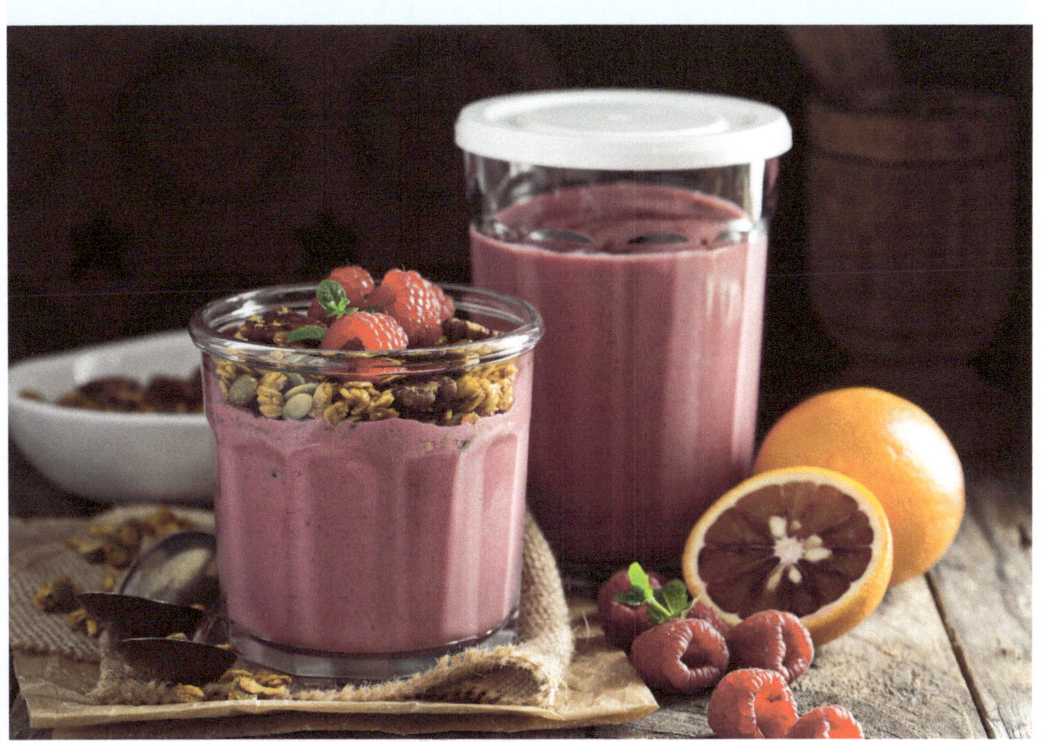

# 09 Apple Cinnamon Smoothie

## INGREDIENTS

- 1 cup diced apples
- 1 banana
- 1 tsp cinnamon
- 1 cup unsweetened almond milk
- 1 scoop vanilla protein powder
- 1 tsp honey

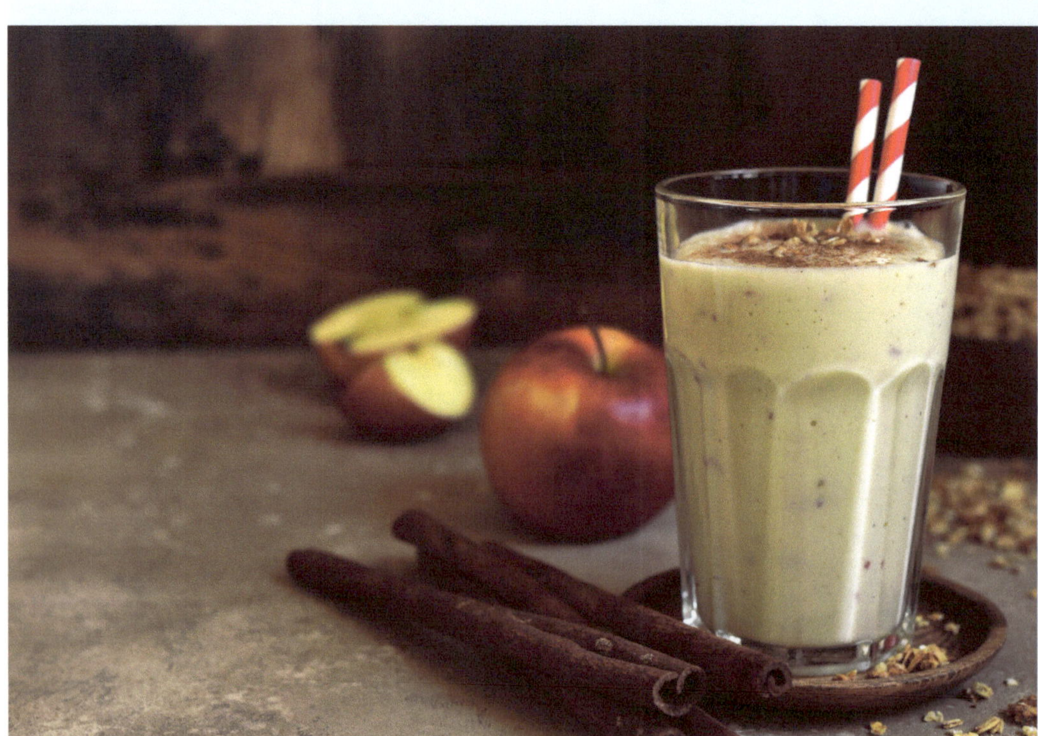

# Acai Bowl Smoothie



## INGREDIENTS

- 1 acai berry packet
- 1 banana
- 1 cup frozen mixed berries
- 1 cup unsweetened almond milk
- 1 scoop vanilla protein powder
- 1 tsp honey

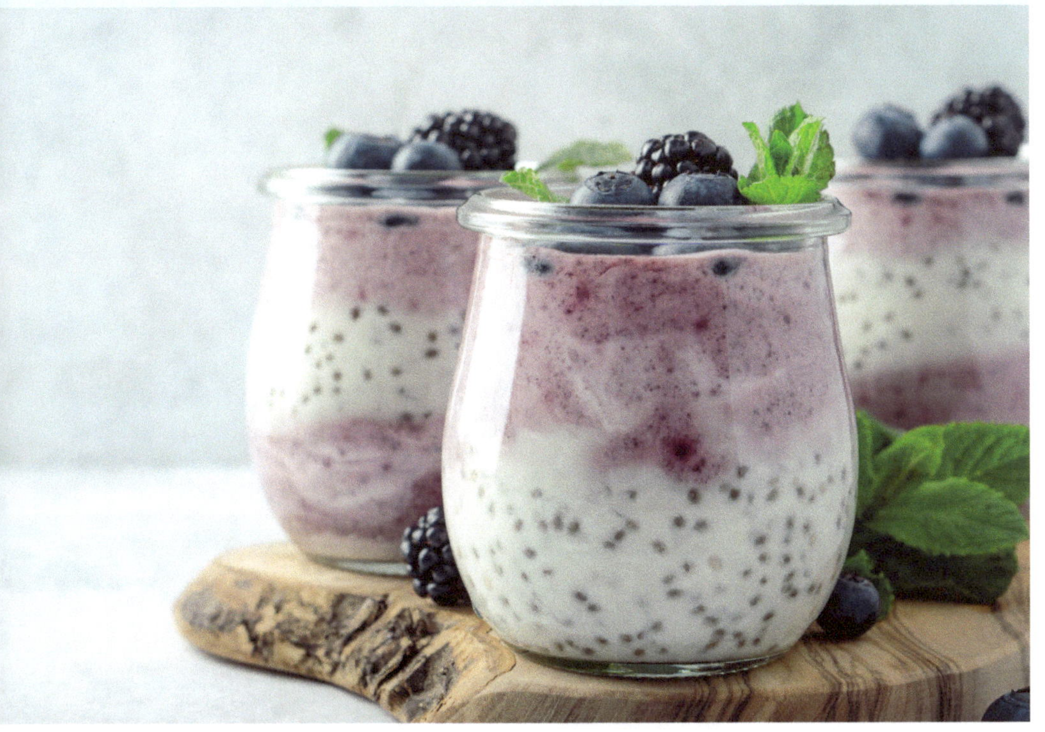

## 11 *Kiwi Lime Smoothie*

## INGREDIENTS

- 2 kiwis, peeled and diced
- 1 lime, juiced
- 1 cup unsweetened almond milk
- 1 scoop vanilla protein powder
- 1 tsp honey

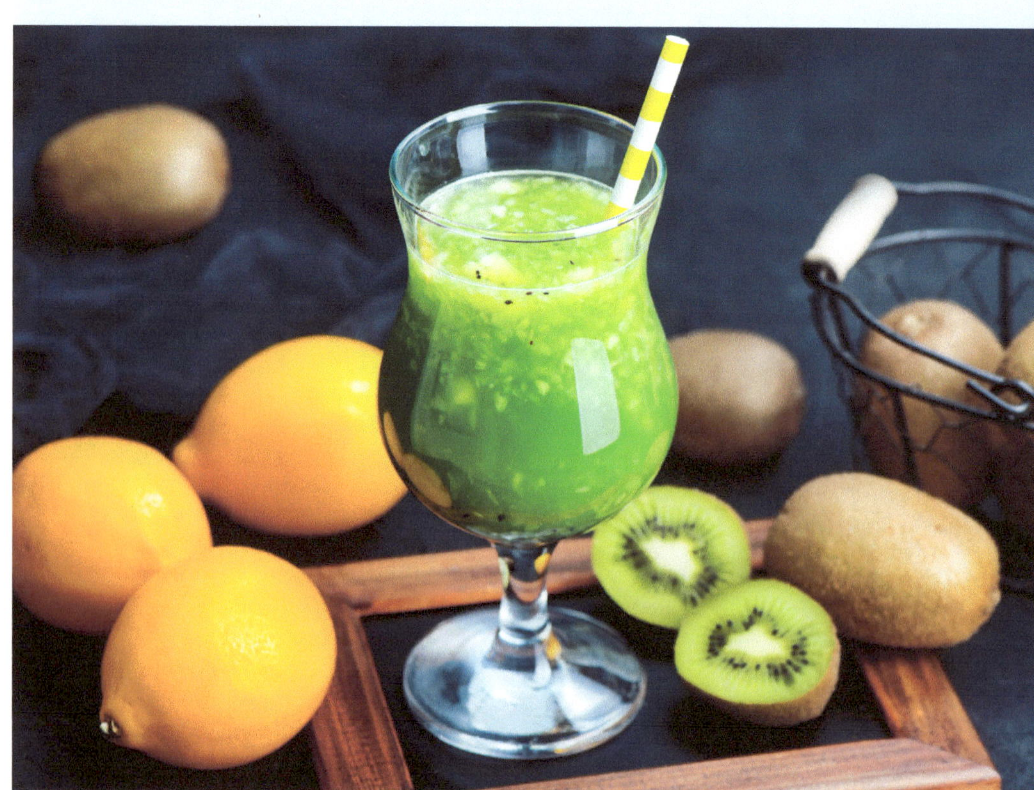

# 12

## Avocado Lime Smoothie

## INGREDIENTS

- 1 avocado, peeled and pitted
- 1 lime, juiced
- 1 cup unsweetened almond milk
- 1 scoop vanilla protein powder
- 1 tsp honey

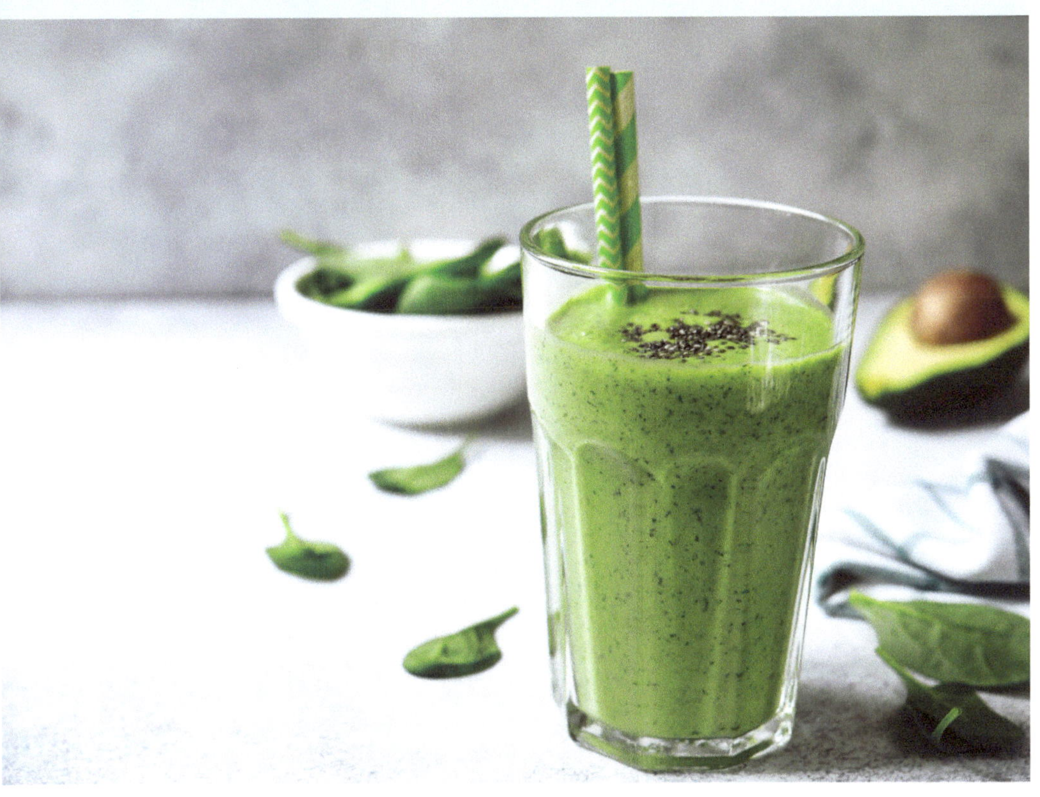

# Cucumber Mint Smoothie

**13**

## INGREDIENTS

- 1 cucumber, peeled and diced
- 1 cup fresh mint leaves
- 1 cup unsweetened almond milk
- 1 scoop vanilla protein powder
- 1 tsp honey

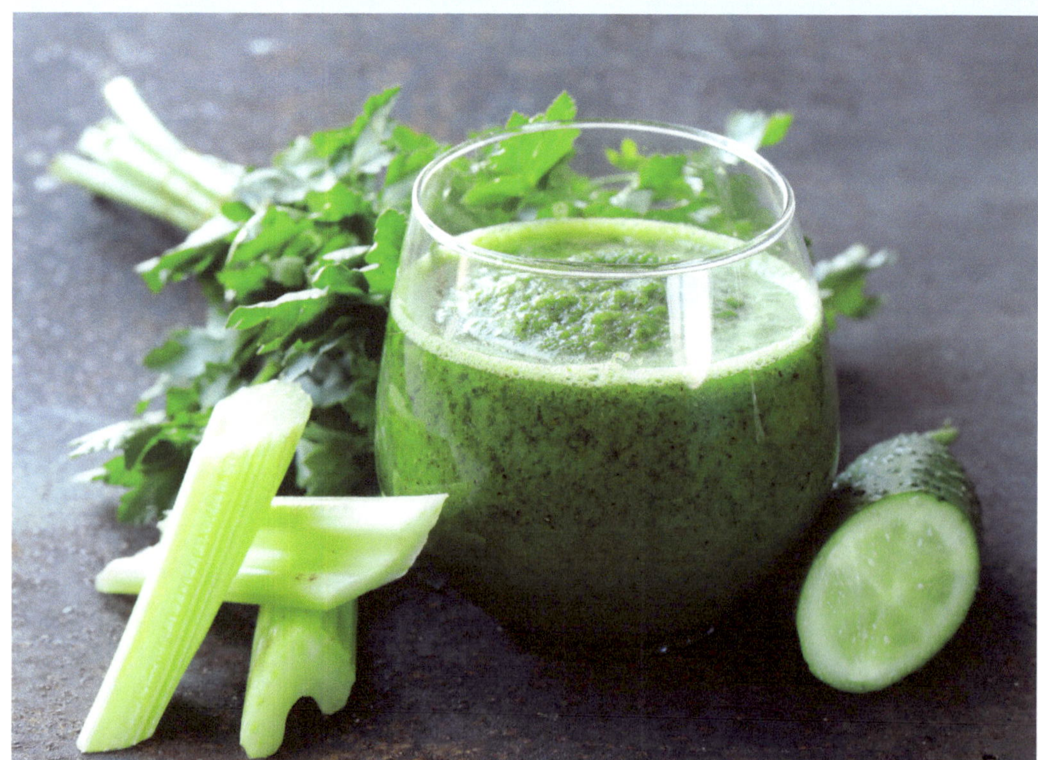

# Beet Berry Smoothie

**14**

## INGREDIENTS

- 1 small beet, peeled and diced
- 1 cup frozen mixed berries
- 1 cup unsweetened almond milk
- 1 scoop vanilla protein powder
- 1 tsp honey

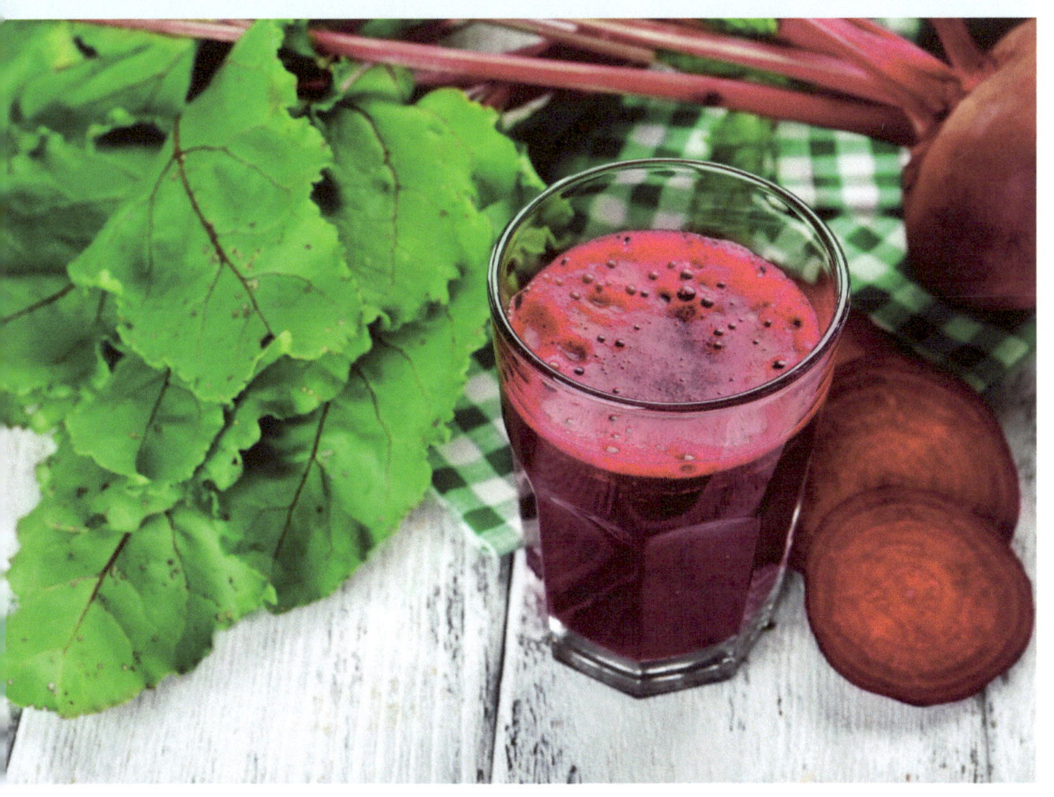

# Carrot Ginger Smoothie

**15**

## INGREDIENTS

- 2 large carrots, peeled and diced
- 1 inch piece of fresh ginger
- 1 cup unsweetened almond milk
- 1 scoop vanilla protein powder
- 1 tsp honey

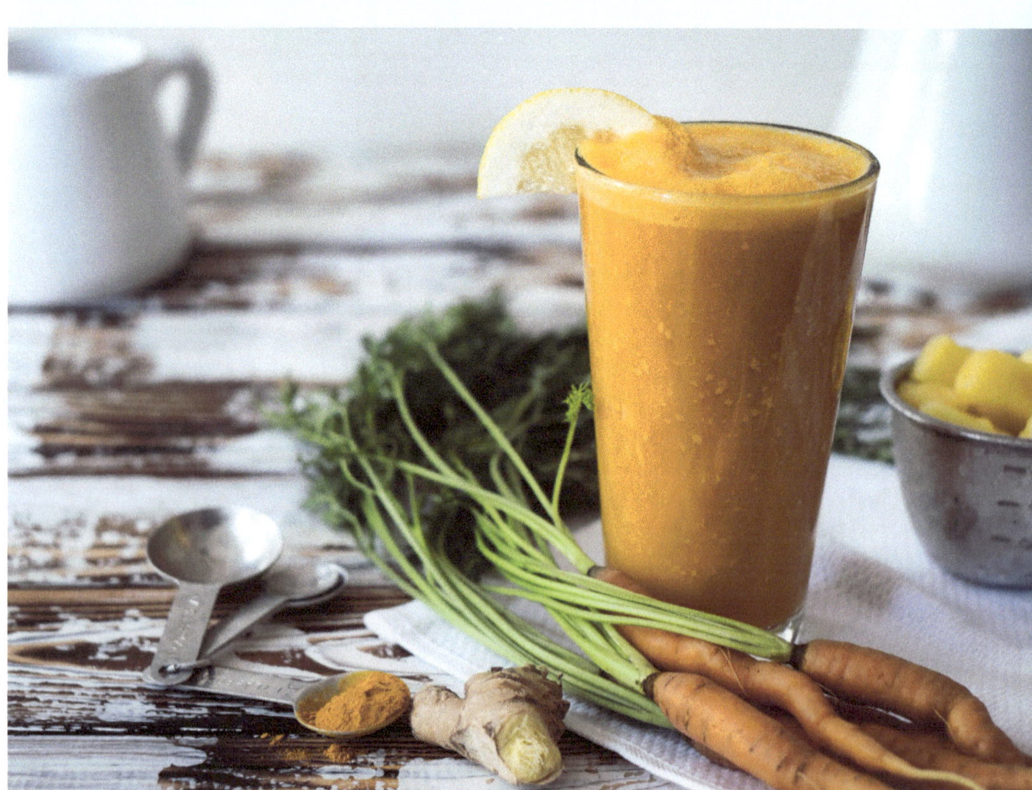

# Spinach Apple Smoothie

## INGREDIENTS

- 2 cups fresh spinach
- 2 apples, peeled and diced
- 1 cup unsweetened almond milk
- 1 scoop vanilla protein powder
- 1 tsp honey

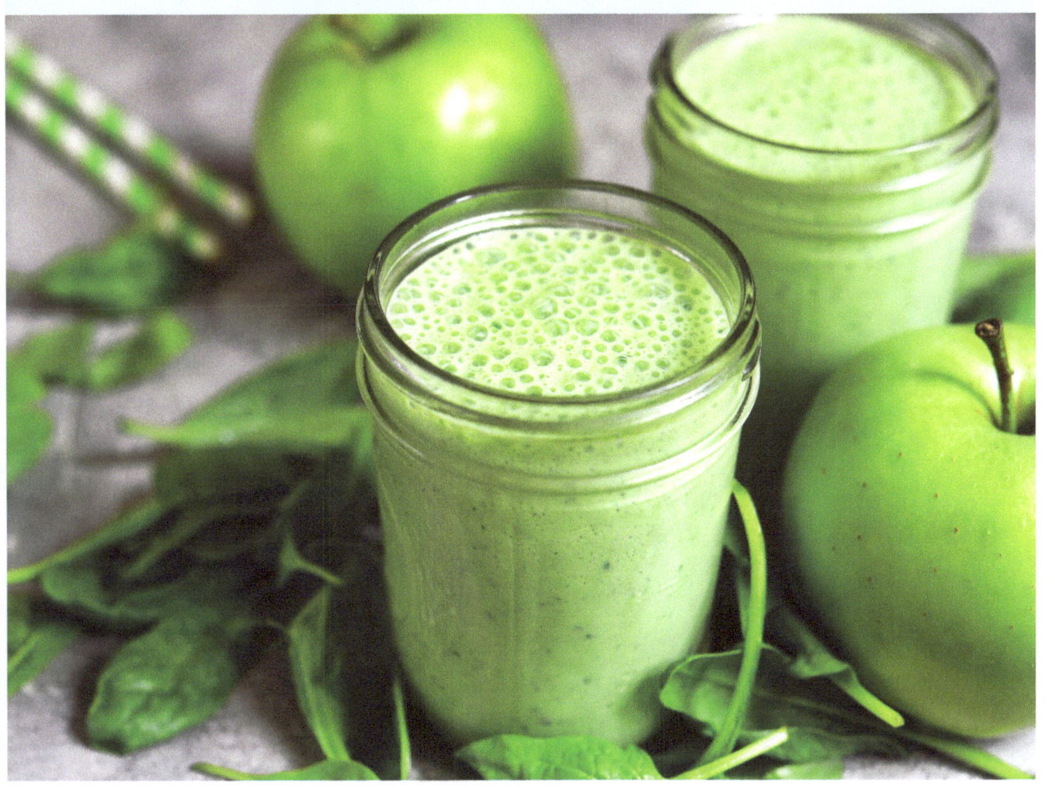

# 17 Mango Banana Smoothie

## INGREDIENTS

- 2 ripe mangoes, peeled and diced
- 2 ripe bananas
- 1 cup unsweetened almond milk
- 1 scoop vanilla protein powder
- 1 tsp honey

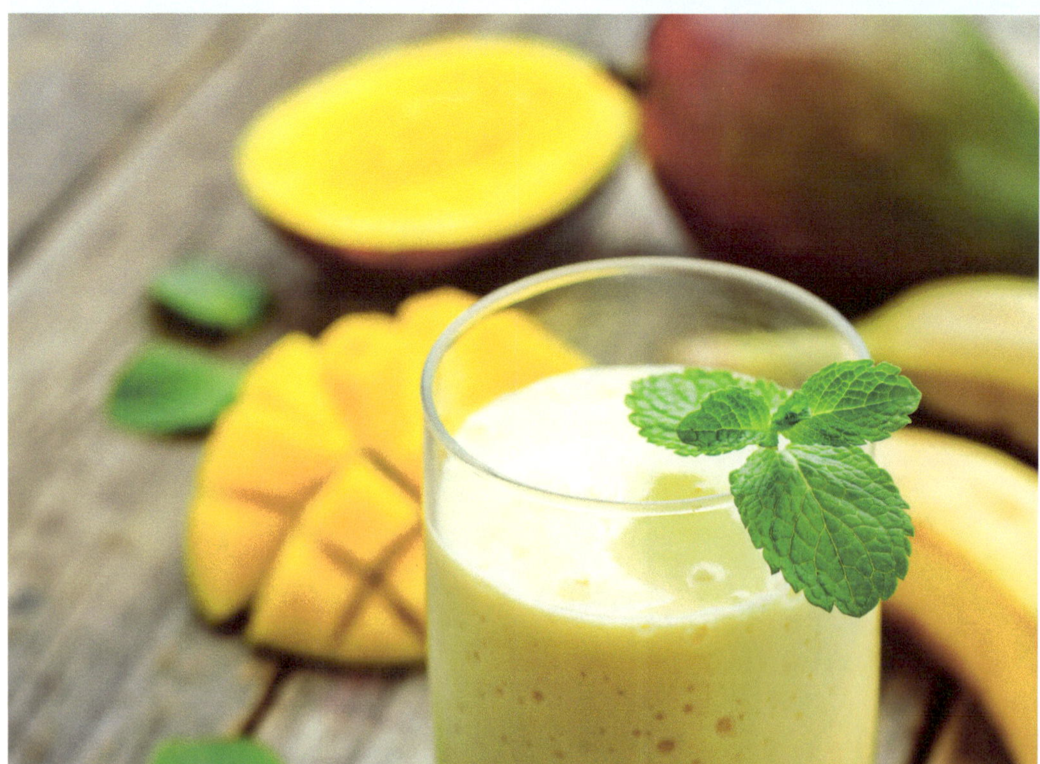

# Blueberry Almond Smoothie

## INGREDIENTS

- 2 cups frozen blueberries
- 1 cup unsweetened almond milk
- 1 scoop vanilla protein powder
- 1 tsp honey
- 1 tbsp almond butter

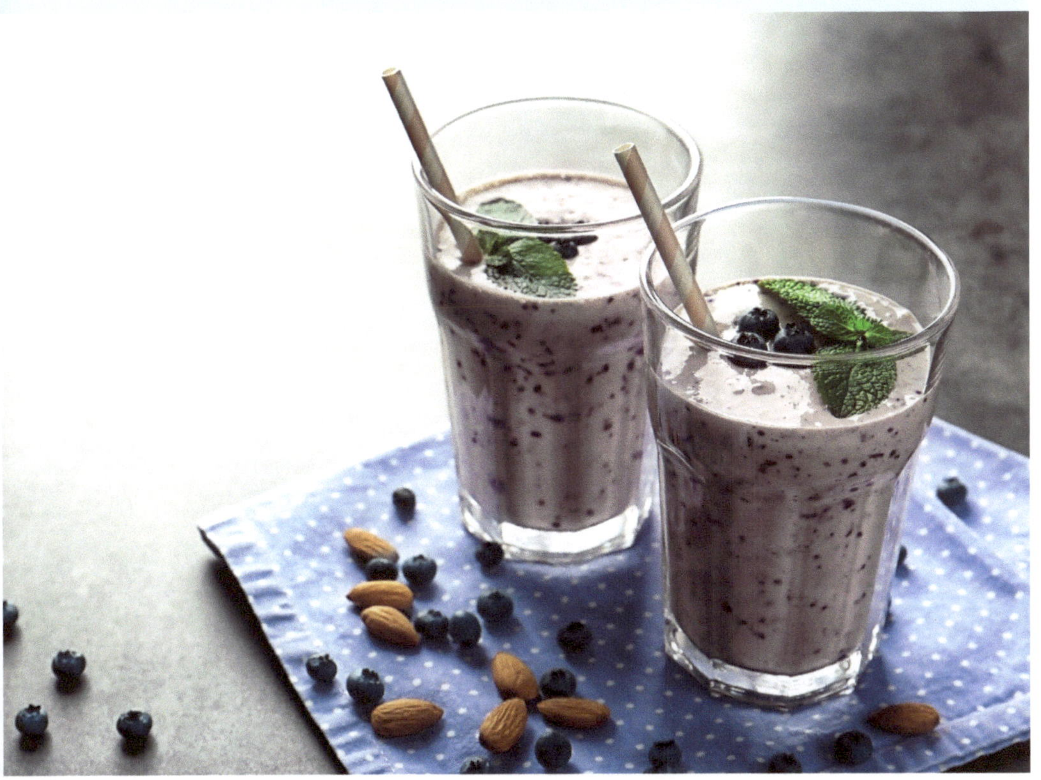

# 19 Peach Ginger Smoothie

## INGREDIENTS

- 2 cups frozen peaches
- 1 inch piece of fresh ginger
- 1 cup unsweetened almond milk
- 1 scoop vanilla protein powder
- 1 tsp honey

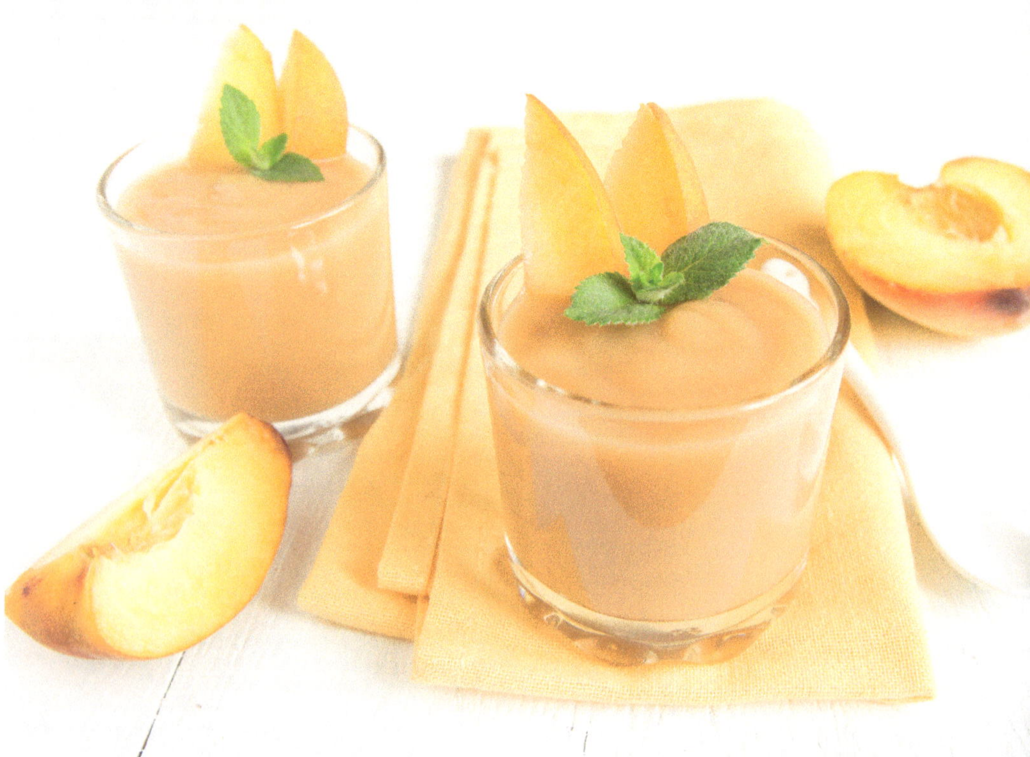

# Raspberry Chia Smoothie

**20**

## INGREDIENTS

- 2 cups frozen raspberries
- 1 cup unsweetened almond milk
- 1 scoop vanilla protein powder
- 1 tsp honey
- 1 tbsp chia seeds

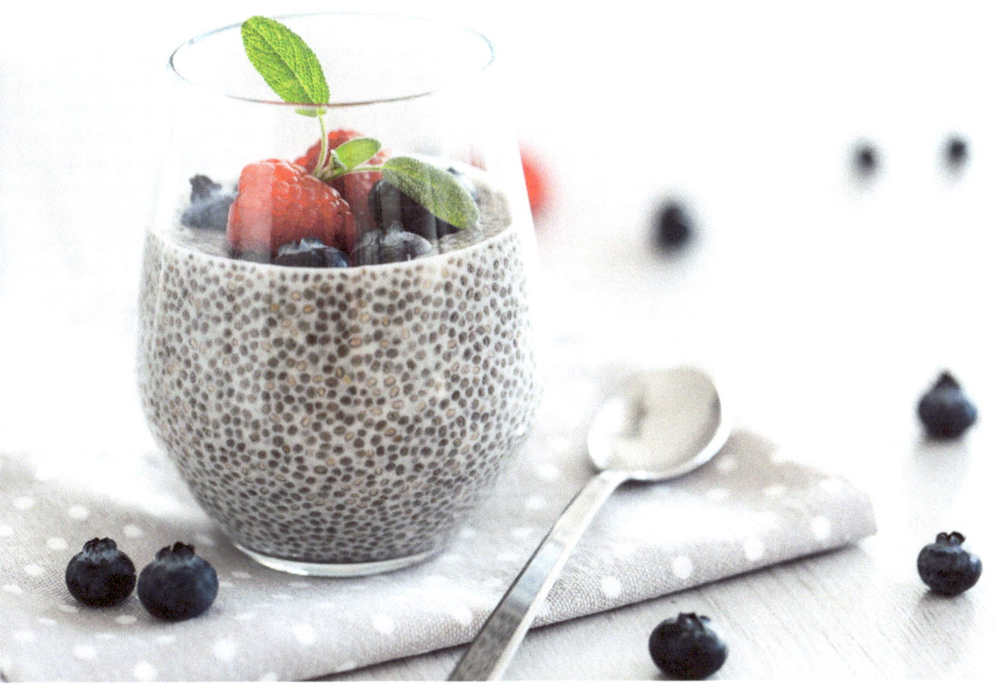

# 21 Chocolate Almond Smoothie

## INGREDIENTS

- 1 scoop chocolate protein powder
- 1 cup unsweetened almond milk
- 1 tsp honey
- 1 tbsp almond butter

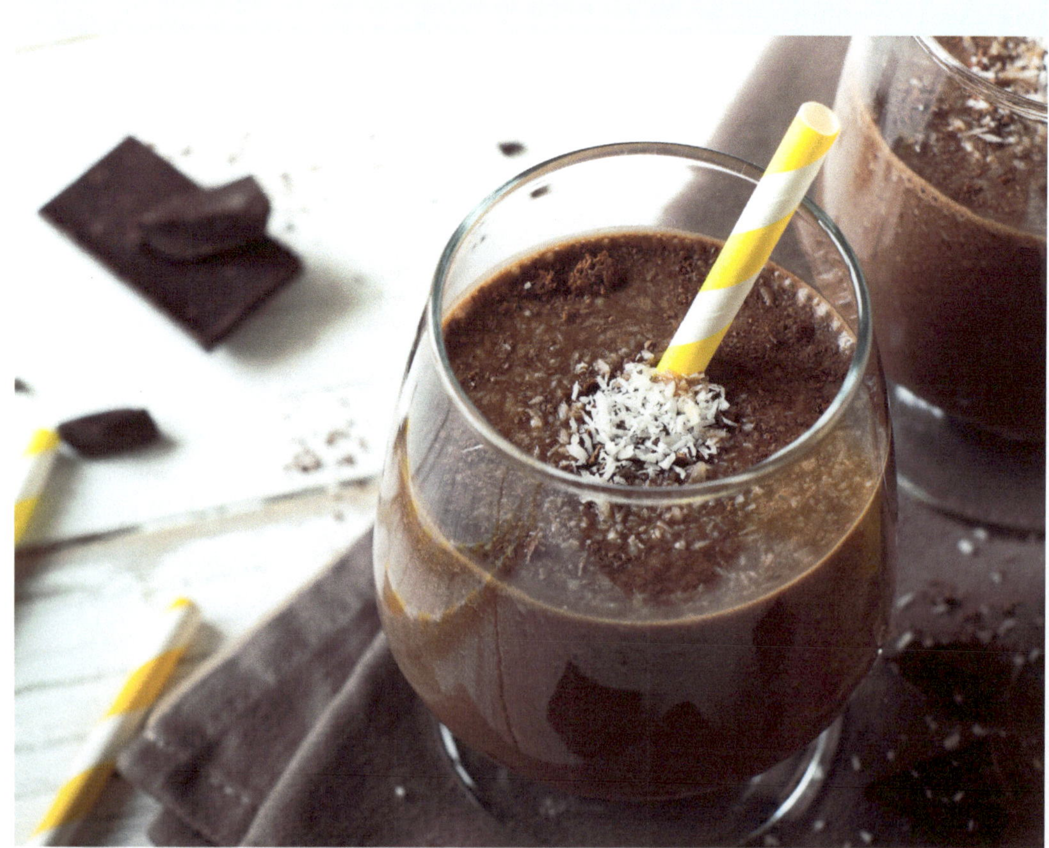

# Avocado Mint Smoothie

**22**

## INGREDIENTS

- 1 ripe avocado
- 1 cup fresh mint leaves
- 1 cup unsweetened almond milk
- 1 scoop vanilla protein powder
- 1 tsp honey

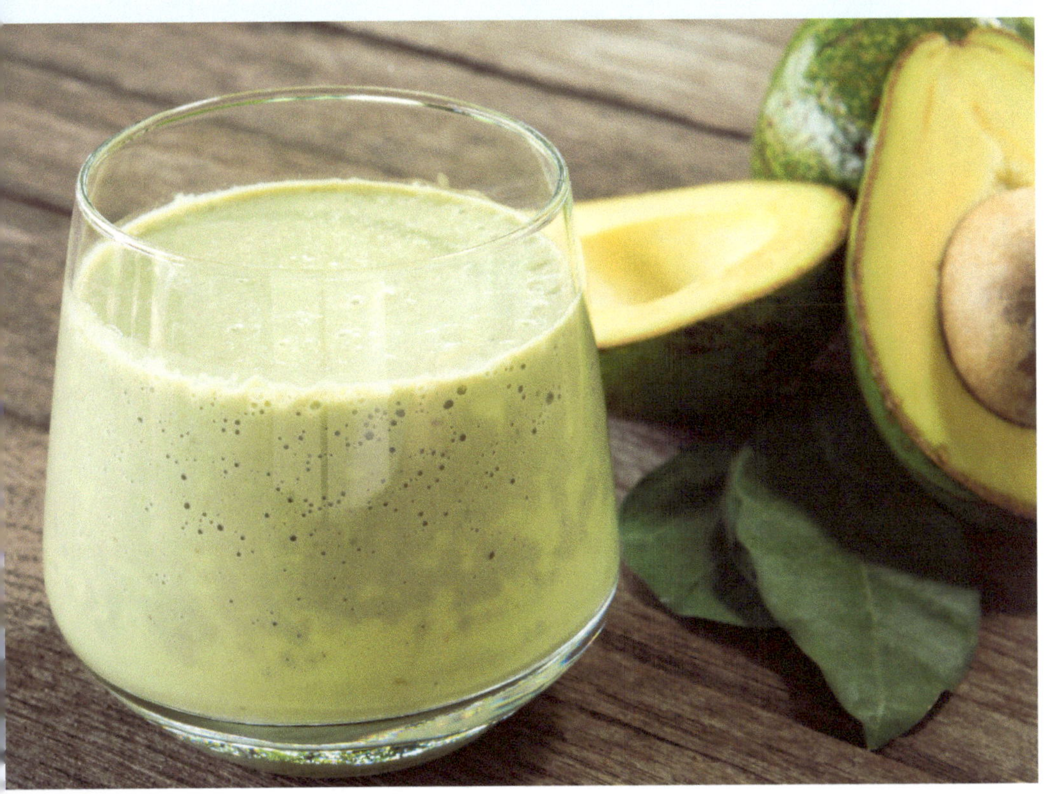

# Carrot Orange Smoothie

## INGREDIENTS

- 2 large carrots, peeled and diced
- 2 medium oranges, peeled and seeded
- 1 cup unsweetened almond milk
- 1 scoop vanilla protein powder
- 1 tsp honey

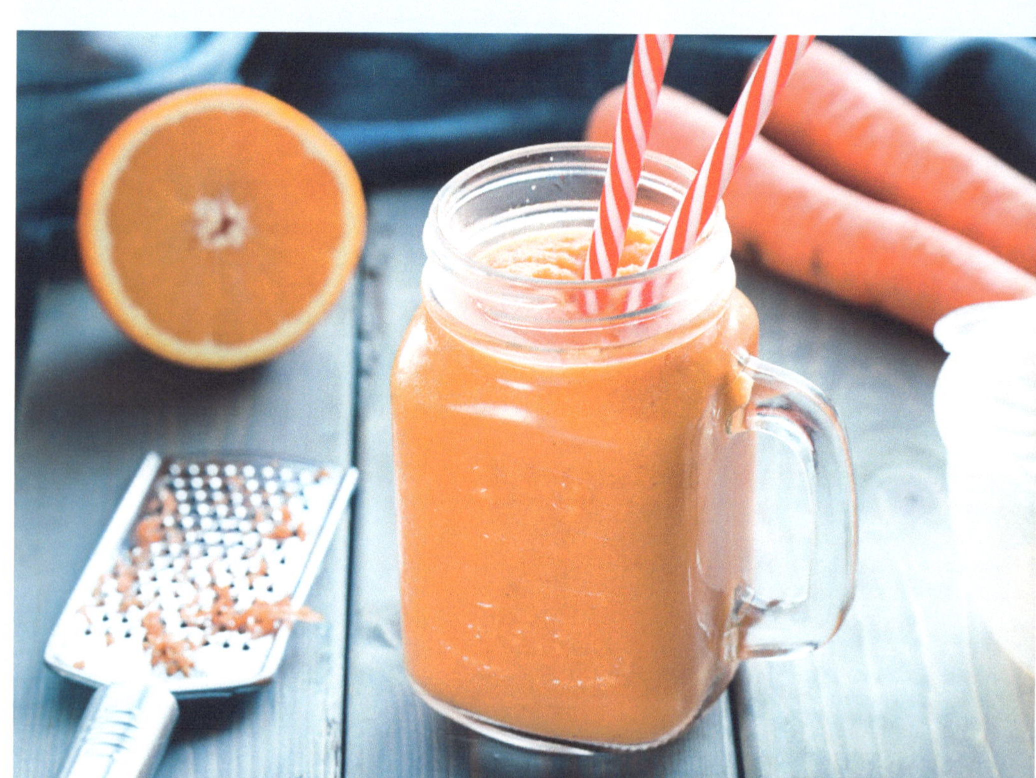

# Cucumber Lime Smoothie

## INGREDIENTS

- 1 large cucumber, peeled and diced
- 1 lime, peeled and seeded
- 1 cup unsweetened almond milk
- 1 scoop vanilla protein powder
- 1 tsp honey

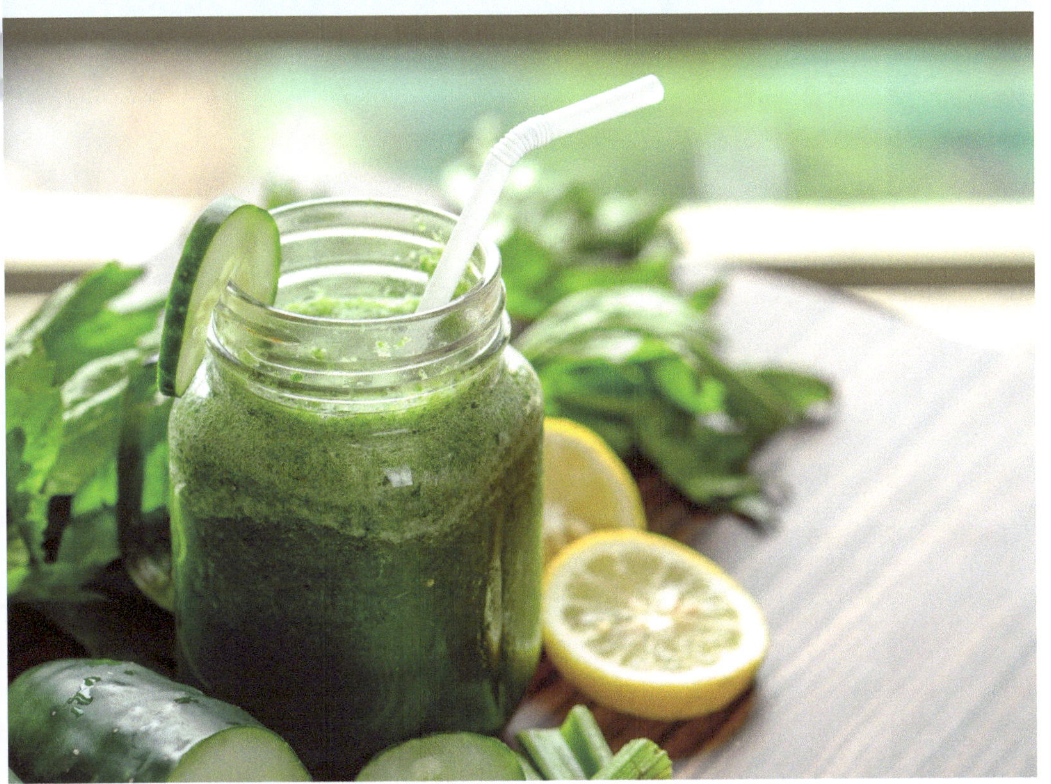

# Blackberry Kale Smoothie



## INGREDIENTS

- 2 cups frozen blackberries
- 2 cups fresh kale leaves
- 1 cup unsweetened almond milk
- 1 scoop vanilla protein powder
- 1 tsp honey

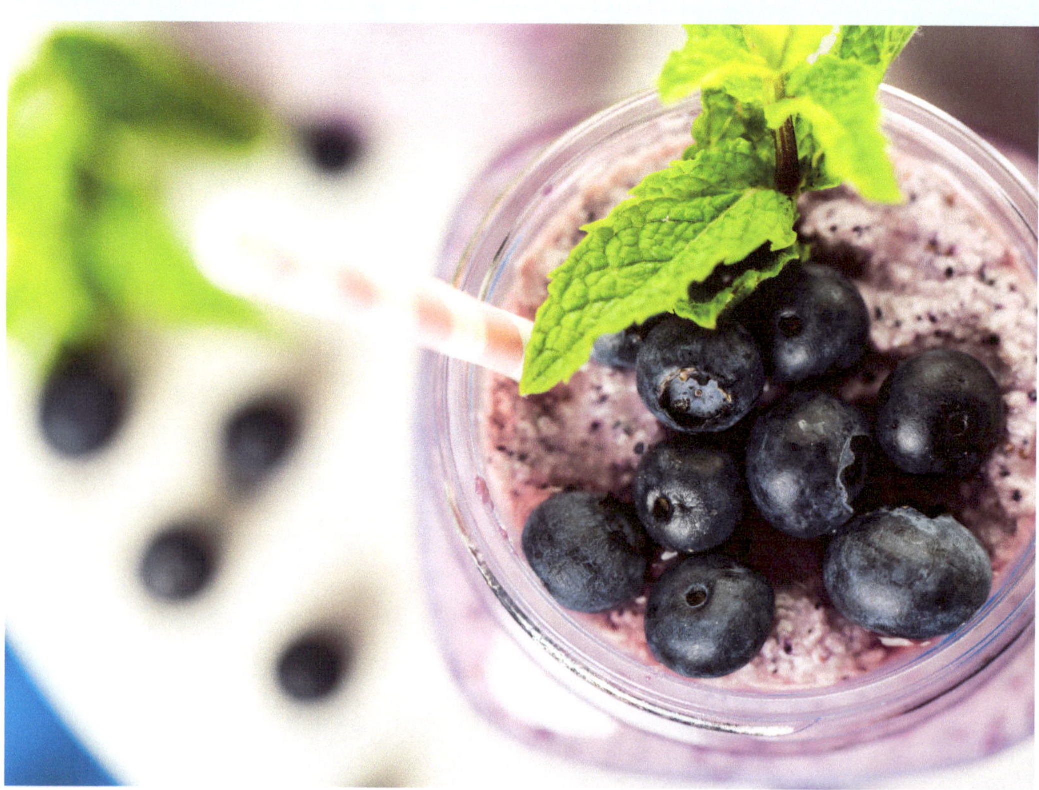

# CONCLUSION

In conclusion, "25 Tasty Smoothies for Weight Loss" is a must-read for anyone who is looking to improve their health and achieve their weight loss goals. Whether you're a seasoned smoothie drinker or new to the world of blended drinks, this book provides all of the information and recipes you need to start enjoying the benefits of healthy and delicious smoothies.

Throughout this book, we have explored the numerous benefits of incorporating smoothies into your diet, including improved digestion, increased energy levels, and weight loss. We have also provided you with 25 easy-to-follow recipes that are specifically designed to help you achieve your weight loss goals while enjoying the taste and convenience of smoothies.

Each recipe in this book is carefully crafted to deliver a delicious and nutritious smoothie that is both easy to make and enjoyable to drink. Whether you're in the mood for something sweet and fruity, or you're looking for a more savory green smoothie, you'll find a recipe that meets your needs and taste preferences. And, because all of the ingredients used in these smoothies are easily accessible, you can make these drinks anytime, anywhere.

# CONCLUSION

So, if you're ready to start your weight loss journey and enjoy the benefits of healthy, delicious smoothies, then grab a blender and let's get started! With 25 tasty smoothie recipes to choose from, you'll never be bored or run out of ideas. Whether you're a busy professional, a student, or simply someone who is looking for a quick and easy way to improve your diet and reach your weight loss goals, this book has got you covered.

In conclusion, "25 Tasty Smoothies for Weight Loss" is a comprehensive guide to the world of healthy and delicious smoothies. It provides all of the information and recipes you need to start enjoying the benefits of smoothies and reaching your weight loss goals. So, don't wait any longer – start blending and enjoying the delicious and nutritious world of smoothies today!

9 7 9 8 3 7 6 5 0 9 2 5 8